Blood Pressure Log

This Book Belongs to

_____

_____

_____

Contact Details

_____

_____

_____

_____

Dedication

This Blood Pressure Log Journal is dedicated to all the people out there who want to track their blood pressure and document their findings in the process.

You are my inspiration for producing books and I'm honored to be a part of keeping all of your blood pressure notes and records organized.

This journal notebook will help you record your details about your blood pressure.

Thoughtfully put together with these sections to record in detail: Date & Time, Weight, Temperature & Blood Pressure.

How to Use this Book

The purpose of this book is to keep all of your Blood Pressure Log notes all in one place. It will help keep you organized.

This Blood Pressure Log will allow you to accurately document every detail about your blood pressure. It's a great way to chart your course through keeping your blood pressure under control.

Here are examples of the prompts for you to fill in and write about your experience in this book:

1. Date & Time

2. Weight

3. Temperature

4. Blood Pressure Reading

Blood Pressure Log

Date	Weight	Temperature	Blood Pressure

Blood Pressure Log

Date	Weight	Temperature	Blood Pressure

Blood Pressure Log

Date	Weight	Temperature	Blood Pressure

Blood Pressure Log

Date	Weight	Temperature	Blood Pressure

Blood Pressure Log

Date	Weight	Temperature	Blood Pressure

Blood Pressure Log

Date	Weight	Temperature	Blood Pressure

Blood Pressure Log

Date	Weight	Temperature	Blood Pressure

Blood Pressure Log

Date	Weight	Temperature	Blood Pressure

Blood Pressure Log

Date	Weight	Temperature	Blood Pressure

Blood Pressure Log

Date	Weight	Temperature	Blood Pressure

Blood Pressure Log

Date	Weight	Temperature	Blood Pressure

Blood Pressure Log

Date	Weight	Temperature	Blood Pressure

Blood Pressure Log

Date	Weight	Temperature	Blood Pressure

Blood Pressure Log

Date	Weight	Temperature	Blood Pressure

Blood Pressure Log

Date	Weight	Temperature	Blood Pressure

Blood Pressure Log

Date	Weight	Temperature	Blood Pressure

Blood Pressure Log

Date	Weight	Temperature	Blood Pressure

Blood Pressure Log

Date	Weight	Temperature	Blood Pressure

Blood Pressure Log

Date	Weight	Temperature	Blood Pressure

Blood Pressure Log

Date	Weight	Temperature	Blood Pressure

Blood Pressure Log

Date	Weight	Temperature	Blood Pressure

Blood Pressure Log

Date	Weight	Temperature	Blood Pressure

Blood Pressure Log

Date	Weight	Temperature	Blood Pressure

Blood Pressure Log

Date	Weight	Temperature	Blood Pressure

Blood Pressure Log

Date	Weight	Temperature	Blood Pressure

Blood Pressure Log

Date	Weight	Temperature	Blood Pressure

Blood Pressure Log

Date	Weight	Temperature	Blood Pressure

Blood Pressure Log

Date	Weight	Temperature	Blood Pressure

Blood Pressure Log

Date	Weight	Temperature	Blood Pressure

Blood Pressure Log

Date	Weight	Temperature	Blood Pressure

Blood Pressure Log

Date	Weight	Temperature	Blood Pressure

Blood Pressure Log

Date	Weight	Temperature	Blood Pressure

Blood Pressure Log

Date	Weight	Temperature	Blood Pressure

Blood Pressure Log

Date	Weight	Temperature	Blood Pressure

Blood Pressure Log

Date	Weight	Temperature	Blood Pressure

Blood Pressure Log

Date	Weight	Temperature	Blood Pressure

Blood Pressure Log

Date	Weight	Temperature	Blood Pressure

Blood Pressure Log

Date	Weight	Temperature	Blood Pressure

Blood Pressure Log

Date	Weight	Temperature	Blood Pressure

Blood Pressure Log

Date	Weight	Temperature	Blood Pressure

Blood Pressure Log

Date	Weight	Temperature	Blood Pressure

Blood Pressure Log

Date	Weight	Temperature	Blood Pressure

Blood Pressure Log

Date	Weight	Temperature	Blood Pressure

Blood Pressure Log

Date	Weight	Temperature	Blood Pressure

Blood Pressure Log

Date	Weight	Temperature	Blood Pressure

Blood Pressure Log

Date	Weight	Temperature	Blood Pressure

Blood Pressure Log

Date	Weight	Temperature	Blood Pressure

Blood Pressure Log

Date	Weight	Temperature	Blood Pressure

Blood Pressure Log

Date	Weight	Temperature	Blood Pressure

Blood Pressure Log

Date	Weight	Temperature	Blood Pressure

Blood Pressure Log

Date	Weight	Temperature	Blood Pressure

Blood Pressure Log

Date	Weight	Temperature	Blood Pressure

Blood Pressure Log

Date	Weight	Temperature	Blood Pressure

Blood Pressure Log

Date	Weight	Temperature	Blood Pressure

Blood Pressure Log

Date	Weight	Temperature	Blood Pressure

Blood Pressure Log

Date	Weight	Temperature	Blood Pressure

Blood Pressure Log

Date	Weight	Temperature	Blood Pressure

Blood Pressure Log

Date	Weight	Temperature	Blood Pressure

Blood Pressure Log

Date	Weight	Temperature	Blood Pressure

Blood Pressure Log

Date	Weight	Temperature	Blood Pressure

Blood Pressure Log

Date	Weight	Temperature	Blood Pressure

Blood Pressure Log

Date	Weight	Temperature	Blood Pressure

Blood Pressure Log

Date	Weight	Temperature	Blood Pressure

Blood Pressure Log

Date	Weight	Temperature	Blood Pressure

Blood Pressure Log

Date	Weight	Temperature	Blood Pressure

Blood Pressure Log

Date	Weight	Temperature	Blood Pressure

Blood Pressure Log

Date	Weight	Temperature	Blood Pressure

Blood Pressure Log

Date	Weight	Temperature	Blood Pressure

Blood Pressure Log

Date	Weight	Temperature	Blood Pressure

Blood Pressure Log

Date	Weight	Temperature	Blood Pressure

Blood Pressure Log

Date	Weight	Temperature	Blood Pressure

Blood Pressure Log

Date	Weight	Temperature	Blood Pressure

Blood Pressure Log

Date	Weight	Temperature	Blood Pressure

Blood Pressure Log

Date	Weight	Temperature	Blood Pressure

Blood Pressure Log

Date	Weight	Temperature	Blood Pressure

Blood Pressure Log

Date	Weight	Temperature	Blood Pressure

Blood Pressure Log

Date	Weight	Temperature	Blood Pressure

Blood Pressure Log

Date	Weight	Temperature	Blood Pressure

Blood Pressure Log

Date	Weight	Temperature	Blood Pressure

Blood Pressure Log

Date	Weight	Temperature	Blood Pressure

Blood Pressure Log

Date	Weight	Temperature	Blood Pressure

Blood Pressure Log

Date	Weight	Temperature	Blood Pressure

Blood Pressure Log

Date	Weight	Temperature	Blood Pressure

Blood Pressure Log

Date	Weight	Temperature	Blood Pressure

Blood Pressure Log

Date	Weight	Temperature	Blood Pressure

Blood Pressure Log

Date	Weight	Temperature	Blood Pressure

Blood Pressure Log

Date	Weight	Temperature	Blood Pressure

Blood Pressure Log

Date	Weight	Temperature	Blood Pressure

Blood Pressure Log

Date	Weight	Temperature	Blood Pressure

Blood Pressure Log

Date	Weight	Temperature	Blood Pressure

Blood Pressure Log

Date	Weight	Temperature	Blood Pressure

Blood Pressure Log

Date	Weight	Temperature	Blood Pressure

Blood Pressure Log

Date	Weight	Temperature	Blood Pressure

Blood Pressure Log

Date	Weight	Temperature	Blood Pressure

Blood Pressure Log

Date	Weight	Temperature	Blood Pressure

Blood Pressure Log

Date	Weight	Temperature	Blood Pressure

Blood Pressure Log

Date	Weight	Temperature	Blood Pressure

Blood Pressure Log

Date	Weight	Temperature	Blood Pressure

Blood Pressure Log

Date	Weight	Temperature	Blood Pressure

Blood Pressure Log

Date	Weight	Temperature	Blood Pressure

www.ingramcontent.com/pod-product-compliance
Lightning Source LLC
Chambersburg PA
CBHW051031030426
42336CB00015B/2827